A Journal of Daily Renewal

A Journal of Daily Renewal

THE COMPANION TO
Make the Connection

BOB GREENE AND
OPRAH WINFREY

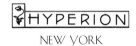
HYPERION
NEW YORK

ISBN 0-7868-8215-8

Designed by Claudyne Bianco Bedell

FIRST EDITION

10 9 8 7 6 5 4 3 2 1

*C*ongratulations on your purchase of *A Journal of Daily Renewal* and on making the commitment to a healthy way of life. *A Journal of Daily Renewal* is the companion to *Make the Connection*, and was developed or you to conveniently record your initial three months of this life-changing pro-ram. The journal should assist you in reaching your goals and in learning about our thoughts and feelings about exercise, eating, and motivation. It also serves as record of what can be a very rewarding journey.

Renewing yourself daily will help you in taking control of your life. Each day, ou should record the basic information regarding your performance of each of the en steps. In addition, each day you should record your thoughts and feelings regard-ng hunger, exercise, eating, thoughts about yourself, thoughts about people in your ife, setbacks, and triumphs—actually, anything you desire. The additional pages in he back of the journal can be used to record your awareness exercises, which are escribed in Chapter Two of *Make the Connection*, and to write about your feelings nd general thoughts before you begin this program and after your initial three nonths of adopting this way of life. Your journal should be as unique as you are.

To help you organize your journal, here's a list of things you can include:

- Your renewal statement for the day (be sure to state your goals and what you will do to work toward them)
- Your general feelings about food, exercise, and life
- Why and when you ate due to stress or emotion
- Any really good events or feelings you had during the day
- Your performance on each of the steps (check off or fill in the following informa-tion)
  How many glasses of water you drank
  Number of fruits and vegetables eaten
  Number of fat grams eaten
  Number of meals and number of snacks eaten
  Number of alcoholic beverages consumed
  Time of your last meal and time you went to sleep
  Minutes of exercise
- Your overall performance rating on how your day went
- Your evening reflection. Reflect on how your day went and how it can be improved tomorrow.

ollowing is a sample journal entry.

DAY 15

Today a new sun rises for me; everything lives, everything is animated, everything seems to speak to me of passion, everything invites me to cherish it.

—Anne De Lenclos

Nov 4 '1995 5:30 Am

I'm still tired from yesterday's 6 mile run. My legs feel like two lead pipes. It's going to be tough trying to maintain the 9:20 pace I've held all week. I'll do my best.

8:17pm I maintained well on the food side. I had 3 low fat cookies instead of 2, but I'm not gonna beat myself up about it. I drank so much water & fuel glasses by the second show I had to stop tape twice for 'p' break

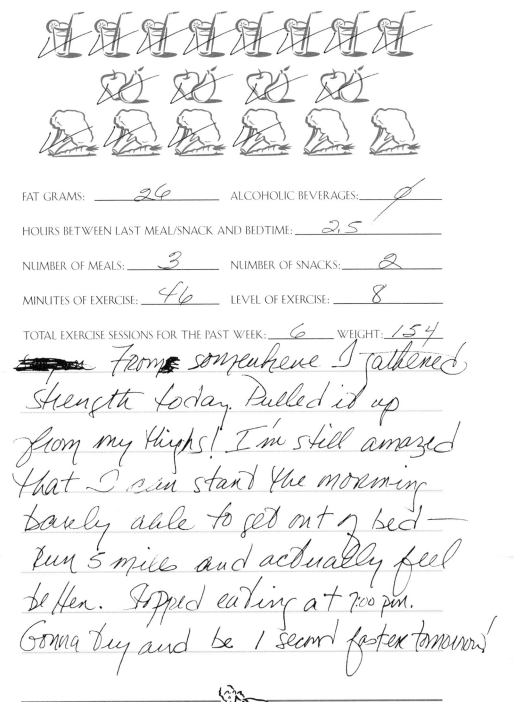

FAT GRAMS: _____26_____ ALCOHOLIC BEVERAGES: _____0_____

HOURS BETWEEN LAST MEAL/SNACK AND BEDTIME: _____2.5_____

NUMBER OF MEALS: _____3_____ NUMBER OF SNACKS: _____2_____

MINUTES OF EXERCISE: _____46_____ LEVEL OF EXERCISE: _____8_____

TOTAL EXERCISE SESSIONS FOR THE PAST WEEK: _____6_____ WEIGHT: _154_

~~From~~ From ~~somewhere~~ somewhere I gathered
strength today. Pulled it up
from my thighs! I'm still amazed
that I can stand the morning
barely able to get out of bed —
run 5 miles and actually feel
better. Stopped eating at 7:00 pm.
Gonna try and be 1 second faster tomorrow!

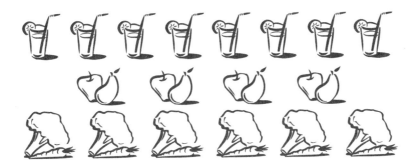

FAT GRAMS: _____   ALCOHOLIC BEVERAGES:_____

HOURS BETWEEN LAST MEAL/SNACK AND BEDTIME: _____

NUMBER OF MEALS: _____   NUMBER OF SNACKS:_____

MINUTES OF EXERCISE: _____   LEVEL OF EXERCISE: _____

DAY 3

The beauty of daily renewal is that no matter how yester-day went, you have the opportunity to improve on it and better yourself today.

—Bob Greene

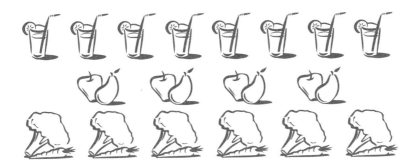

FAT GRAMS: _____ ALCOHOLIC BEVERAGES:_____

HOURS BETWEEN LAST MEAL/SNACK AND BEDTIME: _____

NUMBER OF MEALS: _____ NUMBER OF SNACKS:_____

MINUTES OF EXERCISE: _____ LEVEL OF EXERCISE: _____

DAY 4

It is all about increasing self-confidence, inner strength, and discipline. It is about feeling better on a daily basis, having control over your life, and caring about yourself. Ultimately it is about self-love.

—Bob Greene

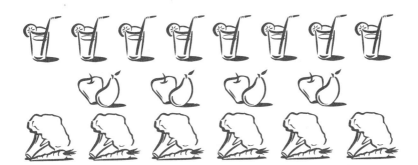

FAT GRAMS: _____ ALCOHOLIC BEVERAGES:_____

HOURS BETWEEN LAST MEAL/SNACK AND BEDTIME: _____

NUMBER OF MEALS: _____ NUMBER OF SNACKS:_____

MINUTES OF EXERCISE: _____ LEVEL OF EXERCISE: _____

_____

_____

_____

_____

_____

_____

_____

DAY 5

But if you have nothing to create, then perhaps you create yourself.

—Carl Jung

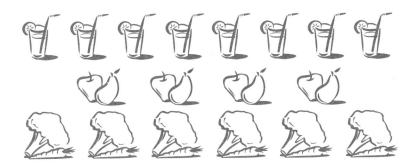

FAT GRAMS: _____ ALCOHOLIC BEVERAGES:_____

HOURS BETWEEN LAST MEAL/SNACK AND BEDTIME: _____

NUMBER OF MEALS: _____ NUMBER OF SNACKS: _____

MINUTES OF EXERCISE: _____ LEVEL OF EXERCISE: _____

_____

_____

_____

_____

_____

_____

_____

_____

DAY 6

Daily renewal is a statement about how you wish your day, and ultimately your life, to unfold. It is your soul speaking to your heart, your heart translating to your mind, and your mind giving your body directions. It is ultimately an expression of self-love!

—Bob Greene

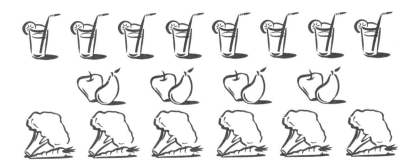

FAT GRAMS: _____ ALCOHOLIC BEVERAGES:_____

HOURS BETWEEN LAST MEAL/SNACK AND BEDTIME: _____

NUMBER OF MEALS: _____ NUMBER OF SNACKS:_____

MINUTES OF EXERCISE: _____ LEVEL OF EXERCISE: _____

_____

_____

_____

_____

_____

_____

_____

_____

_____

DAY 7

As your weight improves, so does your life. And vice versa!

—Bob Greene

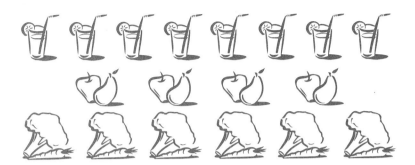

FAT GRAMS: _____ ALCOHOLIC BEVERAGES:_____

HOURS BETWEEN LAST MEAL/SNACK AND BEDTIME: _____

NUMBER OF MEALS: _____ NUMBER OF SNACKS:_____

MINUTES OF EXERCISE: _____ LEVEL OF EXERCISE: _____

DAY 8

Create a positive cycle in your life.

—*Bob Greene*

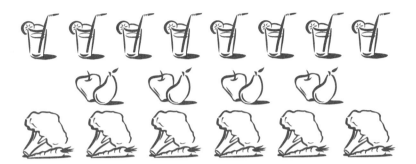

FAT GRAMS: _____ ALCOHOLIC BEVERAGES:_____

HOURS BETWEEN LAST MEAL/SNACK AND BEDTIME: _____

NUMBER OF MEALS: _____ NUMBER OF SNACKS:_____

MINUTES OF EXERCISE: _____ LEVEL OF EXERCISE: _____

TOTAL EXERCISE SESSIONS FOR THE PAST WEEK: _____ WEIGHT:_____

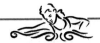

DAY 9

Try to realize, and truly realize, that what stands between you and a different life are matters of responsible choice.

—Gary Zukav

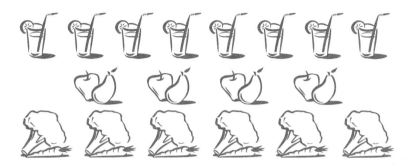

FAT GRAMS: _____ ALCOHOLIC BEVERAGES:_____

HOURS BETWEEN LAST MEAL/SNACK AND BEDTIME: _____

NUMBER OF MEALS: _____ NUMBER OF SNACKS:_____

MINUTES OF EXERCISE: _____ LEVEL OF EXERCISE: _____

_____

_____

_____

_____

_____

_____

_____

_____

DAY 10

Daily renewal is reminding yourself that you are alive and that there is so much you want to accomplish in your life.

–Bob Greene

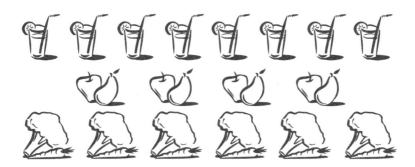

FAT GRAMS: _____ ALCOHOLIC BEVERAGES:_____

HOURS BETWEEN LAST MEAL/SNACK AND BEDTIME: _____

NUMBER OF MEALS: _____ NUMBER OF SNACKS:_____

MINUTES OF EXERCISE: _____ LEVEL OF EXERCISE: _____

DAY 11

If we don't know what we want, we become like a floating balloon. Our direction in life is at the mercy of external forces.

—Bob Greene

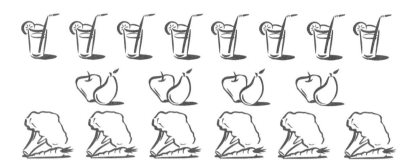

FAT GRAMS: _____ ALCOHOLIC BEVERAGES:_____

HOURS BETWEEN LAST MEAL/SNACK AND BEDTIME: _____

NUMBER OF MEALS: _____ NUMBER OF SNACKS:_____

MINUTES OF EXERCISE: _____ LEVEL OF EXERCISE: _____

_____

_____

_____

_____

_____

_____

_____

DAY 12

If you want your life to come together, you have to start treating yourself better.

—Sara Ban Breathnach

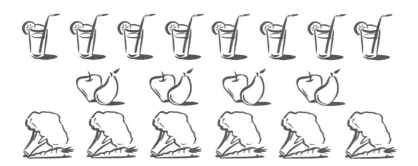

FAT GRAMS: _____ ALCOHOLIC BEVERAGES:_____

HOURS BETWEEN LAST MEAL/SNACK AND BEDTIME: _____

NUMBER OF MEALS: _____ NUMBER OF SNACKS:_____

MINUTES OF EXERCISE: _____ LEVEL OF EXERCISE: _____

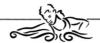

DAY 13

Take responsibility for all that you are and all that you can be.

—Bob Greene

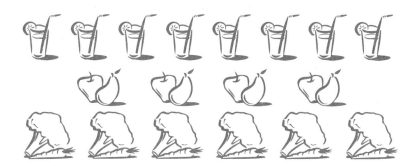

FAT GRAMS: _____ ALCOHOLIC BEVERAGES:_____

HOURS BETWEEN LAST MEAL/SNACK AND BEDTIME: _____

NUMBER OF MEALS: _____ NUMBER OF SNACKS:_____

MINUTES OF EXERCISE: _____ LEVEL OF EXERCISE: _____

DAY 14

Wake up in the morning and announce to yourself: "I want to care more about myself, and I am willing to do what it takes to achieve that. Today, that means I will follow all ten steps. That will be my gift to myself."

—Bob Greene

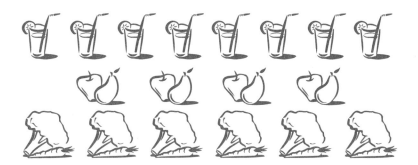

FAT GRAMS: _____ ALCOHOLIC BEVERAGES:_____

HOURS BETWEEN LAST MEAL/SNACK AND BEDTIME: _____

NUMBER OF MEALS: _____ NUMBER OF SNACKS:_____

MINUTES OF EXERCISE: _____ LEVEL OF EXERCISE: _____

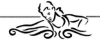

DAY 15

Today a new sun rises for me; everything lives, everything is animated, everything seems to speak to me of passion, everything invites me to cherish it.

—Anne De Lenclos

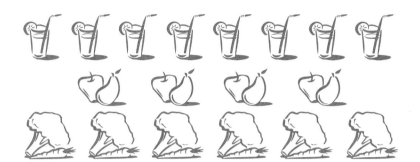

FAT GRAMS: _____ ALCOHOLIC BEVERAGES:_____

HOURS BETWEEN LAST MEAL/SNACK AND BEDTIME: _____

NUMBER OF MEALS: _____ NUMBER OF SNACKS:_____

MINUTES OF EXERCISE: _____ LEVEL OF EXERCISE: _____

TOTAL EXERCISE SESSIONS FOR THE PAST WEEK: _____ WEIGHT:_____

_____

_____

_____

_____

_____

_____

_____

DAY 16

Food is a true pleasure . . . one to be enjoyed and experienced.

—*Bob Greene*

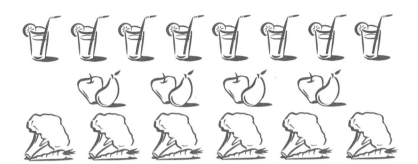

FAT GRAMS: _____ ALCOHOLIC BEVERAGES:_____

HOURS BETWEEN LAST MEAL/SNACK AND BEDTIME: _____

NUMBER OF MEALS: _____ NUMBER OF SNACKS:_____

MINUTES OF EXERCISE: _____ LEVEL OF EXERCISE: _____

DAY 17

Any goal worth reaching always requires hard work.

—Bob Greene

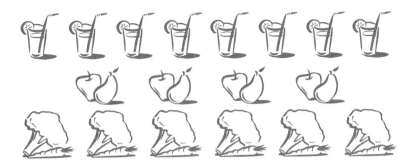

FAT GRAMS: _____ ALCOHOLIC BEVERAGES:_____

HOURS BETWEEN LAST MEAL/SNACK AND BEDTIME: _____

NUMBER OF MEALS: _____ NUMBER OF SNACKS:_____

MINUTES OF EXERCISE: _____ LEVEL OF EXERCISE: _____

_____

_____

_____

_____

_____

_____

_____

_____

DAY 18

You have to change your perception. It's not about weight—it's about caring for yourself on a daily basis. Renew! Renew! Renew!

—Oprah Winfrey

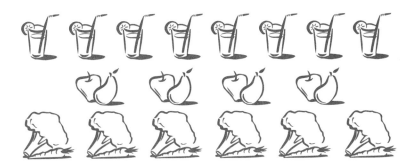

FAT GRAMS: _____ ALCOHOLIC BEVERAGES:_____

HOURS BETWEEN LAST MEAL/SNACK AND BEDTIME: _____

NUMBER OF MEALS: _____ NUMBER OF SNACKS:_____

MINUTES OF EXERCISE: _____ LEVEL OF EXERCISE: _____

_____

_____

_____

_____

_____

_____

_____

_____

_____

DAY 19

Health is the vital principle of bliss, and exercise, of health.

—James Thompson

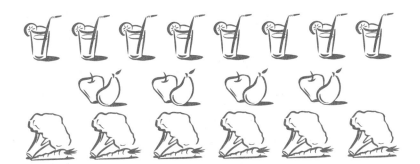

FAT GRAMS: _____ ALCOHOLIC BEVERAGES:_____

HOURS BETWEEN LAST MEAL/SNACK AND BEDTIME: _____

NUMBER OF MEALS: _____ NUMBER OF SNACKS:_____

MINUTES OF EXERCISE: _____ LEVEL OF EXERCISE: _____

_____

_____

_____

_____

_____

_____

_____

_____

DAY 20

Only when you have self-awareness can you achieve self-acceptance.

—Bob Greene

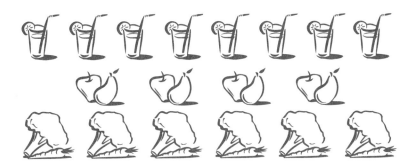

FAT GRAMS: _____ ALCOHOLIC BEVERAGES:_____

HOURS BETWEEN LAST MEAL/SNACK AND BEDTIME: _____

NUMBER OF MEALS: _____ NUMBER OF SNACKS:_____

MINUTES OF EXERCISE: _____ LEVEL OF EXERCISE: _____

DAY 21

Only when you have accepted yourself can you experience self-love.

—Bob Greene

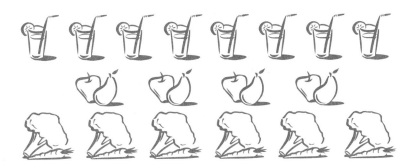

FAT GRAMS: _____ ALCOHOLIC BEVERAGES:_____

HOURS BETWEEN LAST MEAL/SNACK AND BEDTIME: _____

NUMBER OF MEALS: _____ NUMBER OF SNACKS:_____

MINUTES OF EXERCISE: _____ LEVEL OF EXERCISE: _____

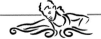

DAY 22

Self-awareness, self-acceptance, and self-love are lifelong processes.

—Bob Greene

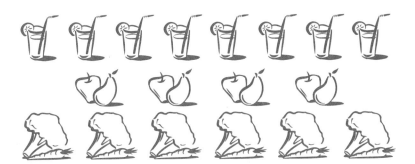

FAT GRAMS: _____ ALCOHOLIC BEVERAGES:_____

HOURS BETWEEN LAST MEAL/SNACK AND BEDTIME: _____

NUMBER OF MEALS: _____ NUMBER OF SNACKS:_____

MINUTES OF EXERCISE: _____ LEVEL OF EXERCISE: _____

TOTAL EXERCISE SESSIONS FOR THE PAST WEEK: _____ WEIGHT:_____

_____

_____

_____

_____

_____

_____

_____

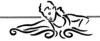

DAY 23

Self-awareness means facing the facts about yourself, both good and bad. Denial is a detour that leads you to nowhere.

—Bob Greene

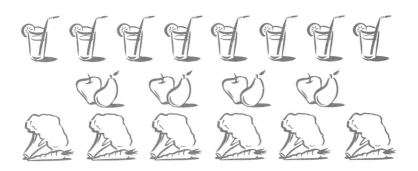

FAT GRAMS: _____ ALCOHOLIC BEVERAGES:_____

HOURS BETWEEN LAST MEAL/SNACK AND BEDTIME: _____

NUMBER OF MEALS: _____ NUMBER OF SNACKS:_____

MINUTES OF EXERCISE: _____ LEVEL OF EXERCISE: _____

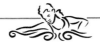

DAY 24

I will tell you what I learned for myself. For me a long, five- or six-mile walk helps. And one must go alone and every day.

—Brenda Ueland

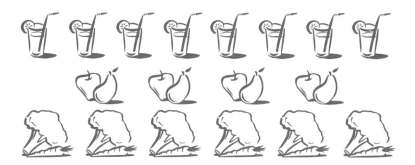

FAT GRAMS: _____ ALCOHOLIC BEVERAGES:_____

HOURS BETWEEN LAST MEAL/SNACK AND BEDTIME: _____

NUMBER OF MEALS: _____ NUMBER OF SNACKS:_____

MINUTES OF EXERCISE: _____ LEVEL OF EXERCISE: _____

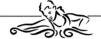

DAY 25

Look to your health; and if you have it, praise God, and value it next to a good conscience; for health is the second blessing we mortals are capable of; a blessing money cannot buy.

—Izaak Walton

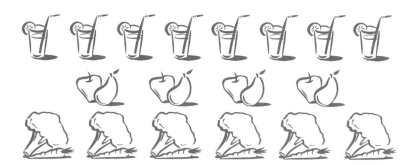

FAT GRAMS: _____ ALCOHOLIC BEVERAGES:_____

HOURS BETWEEN LAST MEAL/SNACK AND BEDTIME: _____

NUMBER OF MEALS: _____ NUMBER OF SNACKS:_____

MINUTES OF EXERCISE: _____ LEVEL OF EXERCISE: _____

_____

_____

_____

_____

_____

_____

_____

_____

_____

_____

DAY 26

Your body gives you what it has.

—Bob Greene

_____

_____

_____

_____

_____

_____

_____

_____

_____

_____

_____

_____

_____

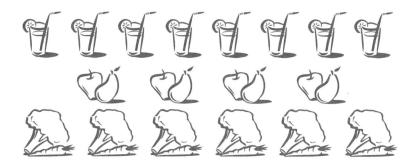

FAT GRAMS: _____ ALCOHOLIC BEVERAGES:_____

HOURS BETWEEN LAST MEAL/SNACK AND BEDTIME: _____

NUMBER OF MEALS: _____ NUMBER OF SNACKS:_____

MINUTES OF EXERCISE: _____ LEVEL OF EXERCISE: _____

_____

_____

_____

_____

_____

_____

_____

_____

DAY 27

The body is shaped, disciplined, honored, and in time, trusted.

—Martha Graham

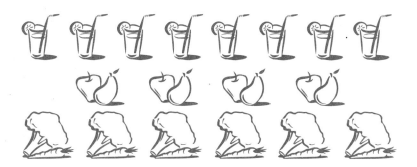

FAT GRAMS: _____ ALCOHOLIC BEVERAGES:_____

HOURS BETWEEN LAST MEAL/SNACK AND BEDTIME: _____

NUMBER OF MEALS: _____ NUMBER OF SNACKS:_____

MINUTES OF EXERCISE: _____ LEVEL OF EXERCISE: _____

DAY 28

Our deepest fear is not that we are inadequate. Our deepest fear is that we are powerful beyond measure.

— Marianne Williamson

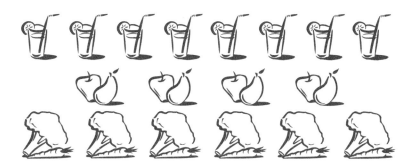

FAT GRAMS: _____ ALCOHOLIC BEVERAGES:_____

HOURS BETWEEN LAST MEAL/SNACK AND BEDTIME: _____

NUMBER OF MEALS: _____ NUMBER OF SNACKS:_____

MINUTES OF EXERCISE: _____ LEVEL OF EXERCISE: _____

DAY 29

Working out allows you to be more aware.

—Oprah Winfrey

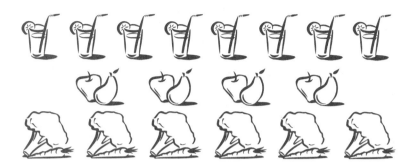

FAT GRAMS: _____ ALCOHOLIC BEVERAGES:_____

HOURS BETWEEN LAST MEAL/SNACK AND BEDTIME: _____

NUMBER OF MEALS: _____ NUMBER OF SNACKS:_____

MINUTES OF EXERCISE: _____ LEVEL OF EXERCISE: _____

TOTAL EXERCISE SESSIONS FOR THE PAST WEEK: _____ WEIGHT:_____

DAY 30

Things do not change, we change.

—Henry David Thoreau

FAT GRAMS: _____ ALCOHOLIC BEVERAGES: _____

HOURS BETWEEN LAST MEAL/SNACK AND BEDTIME: _____

NUMBER OF MEALS: _____ NUMBER OF SNACKS: _____

MINUTES OF EXERCISE: _____ LEVEL OF EXERCISE: _____

DAY 31

Any little bit of experimenting in self-nurturance is very frightening for most of us.

—Julia Cameron

FAT GRAMS: _____ ALCOHOLIC BEVERAGES: _____

HOURS BETWEEN LAST MEAL/SNACK AND BEDTIME: _____

NUMBER OF MEALS: _____ NUMBER OF SNACKS: _____

MINUTES OF EXERCISE: _____ LEVEL OF EXERCISE: _____

DAY 32

To be successful at long-term weight loss, you must be both consistent and patient.

—Bob Greene

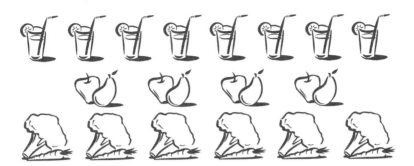

FAT GRAMS: _____ ALCOHOLIC BEVERAGES: _____

HOURS BETWEEN LAST MEAL/SNACK AND BEDTIME: _____

NUMBER OF MEALS: _____ NUMBER OF SNACKS: _____

MINUTES OF EXERCISE: _____ LEVEL OF EXERCISE: _____

DAY 33

For years I'd dieted and occasionally got moving, but I wasn't moving enough. I was never consistent.

—Oprah Winfrey

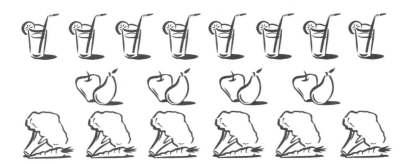

FAT GRAMS: _____ ALCOHOLIC BEVERAGES:_____

HOURS BETWEEN LAST MEAL/SNACK AND BEDTIME: _____

NUMBER OF MEALS: _____ NUMBER OF SNACKS:_____

MINUTES OF EXERCISE: _____ LEVEL OF EXERCISE: _____

DAY 34

When the stomach is full, it is easy to talk of fasting.
—Saint Jerome

FAT GRAMS: _____ ALCOHOLIC BEVERAGES:_____

HOURS BETWEEN LAST MEAL/SNACK AND BEDTIME: _____

NUMBER OF MEALS: _____ NUMBER OF SNACKS:_____

MINUTES OF EXERCISE: _____ LEVEL OF EXERCISE: _____

_____

_____

_____

_____

_____

_____

_____

_____

_____

DAY 35

Live now, believe me, wait not till tomorrow; gather the roses of life today.

—Pierre de Ronsard

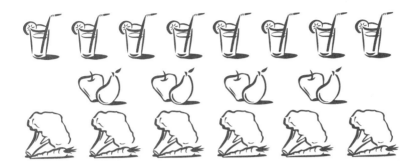

FAT GRAMS: _____ ALCOHOLIC BEVERAGES:_____

HOURS BETWEEN LAST MEAL/SNACK AND BEDTIME: _____

NUMBER OF MEALS: _____ NUMBER OF SNACKS:_____

MINUTES OF EXERCISE: _____ LEVEL OF EXERCISE: _____

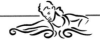

DAY 36

A man should always consider how much he has more than he wants; and secondly, how much more unhappy he might be than he really is.

—Joseph Addison

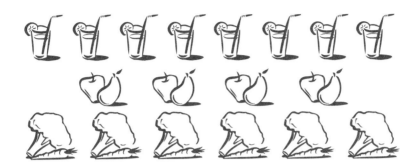

FAT GRAMS: _____ ALCOHOLIC BEVERAGES:_____

HOURS BETWEEN LAST MEAL/SNACK AND BEDTIME: _____

NUMBER OF MEALS: _____ NUMBER OF SNACKS:_____

MINUTES OF EXERCISE: _____ LEVEL OF EXERCISE: _____

TOTAL EXERCISE SESSIONS FOR THE PAST WEEK: _____ WEIGHT:_____

_____

_____

_____

_____

_____

_____

_____

DAY 37

Seek not outside yourself, heaven is within.

—Mary Lou Cook

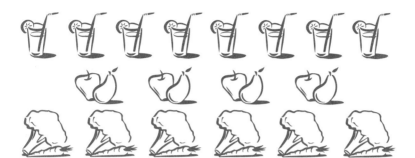

FAT GRAMS: _____ ALCOHOLIC BEVERAGES:_____

HOURS BETWEEN LAST MEAL/SNACK AND BEDTIME: _____

NUMBER OF MEALS: _____ NUMBER OF SNACKS:_____

MINUTES OF EXERCISE: _____ LEVEL OF EXERCISE: _____

_____

_____

_____

_____

_____

_____

_____

_____

DAY 38

Always be a first-rate version of yourself, instead of a second-rate version of somebody else.

—Judy Garland

FAT GRAMS: _____ ALCOHOLIC BEVERAGES:_____

HOURS BETWEEN LAST MEAL/SNACK AND BEDTIME: _____

NUMBER OF MEALS: _____ NUMBER OF SNACKS:_____

MINUTES OF EXERCISE: _____ LEVEL OF EXERCISE: _____

DAY 39

We are the hero of our own story.

—Mary McCarthy

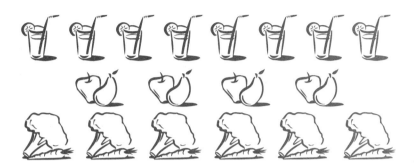

FAT GRAMS: _____ ALCOHOLIC BEVERAGES:_____

HOURS BETWEEN LAST MEAL/SNACK AND BEDTIME: _____

NUMBER OF MEALS: _____ NUMBER OF SNACKS: _____

MINUTES OF EXERCISE: _____ LEVEL OF EXERCISE: _____

_____

_____

_____

_____

_____

_____

_____

_____

DAY 40

I am not one of those people who claims they love to exercise. I simply love all that it does for me.

—Oprah Winfrey

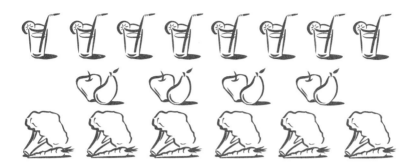

FAT GRAMS: _____ ALCOHOLIC BEVERAGES:_____

HOURS BETWEEN LAST MEAL/SNACK AND BEDTIME: _____

NUMBER OF MEALS: _____ NUMBER OF SNACKS:_____

MINUTES OF EXERCISE: _____ LEVEL OF EXERCISE: _____

DAY 41

It is only by believing, hoping, loving, and doing that man finds joy.

—John Lancaster Spalding

FAT GRAMS: _____ ALCOHOLIC BEVERAGES: _____

HOURS BETWEEN LAST MEAL/SNACK AND BEDTIME: _____

NUMBER OF MEALS: _____ NUMBER OF SNACKS: _____

MINUTES OF EXERCISE: _____ LEVEL OF EXERCISE: _____

DAY 42

Self-reverence, self-knowledge, self-control. These three alone lead life to sovereign power.

—Alfred, Lord Tennyson

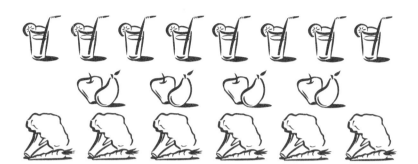

FAT GRAMS: _____ ALCOHOLIC BEVERAGES: _____

HOURS BETWEEN LAST MEAL/SNACK AND BEDTIME: _____

NUMBER OF MEALS: _____ NUMBER OF SNACKS: _____

MINUTES OF EXERCISE: _____ LEVEL OF EXERCISE: _____

DAY 43

The most important part is to understand that it's not as much about the weight as it is about making the connection.

—Oprah Winfrey

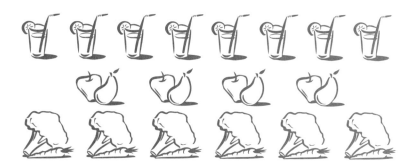

FAT GRAMS: _____ ALCOHOLIC BEVERAGES:_____

HOURS BETWEEN LAST MEAL/SNACK AND BEDTIME: _____

NUMBER OF MEALS: _____ NUMBER OF SNACKS:_____

MINUTES OF EXERCISE: _____ LEVEL OF EXERCISE: _____

TOTAL EXERCISE SESSIONS FOR THE PAST WEEK: _____ WEIGHT:_____

_____

_____

_____

_____

_____

_____

_____

_____

DAY 44

You will know you have made the connection when you care enough about yourself that you would never consider doing anything outside your best interest.

—Bob Greene

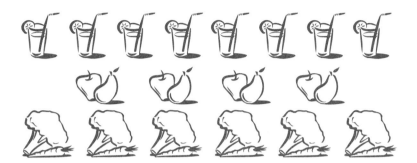

FAT GRAMS: _____ ALCOHOLIC BEVERAGES: _____

HOURS BETWEEN LAST MEAL/SNACK AND BEDTIME: _____

NUMBER OF MEALS: _____ NUMBER OF SNACKS: _____

MINUTES OF EXERCISE: _____ LEVEL OF EXERCISE: _____

_____

_____

_____

_____

_____

_____

_____

_____

DAY 45

When you make the connection, your life will change.

—Bob Greene

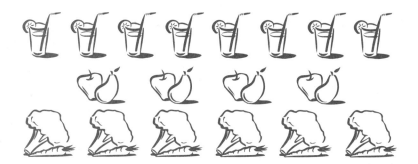

FAT GRAMS: _____ ALCOHOLIC BEVERAGES:_____

HOURS BETWEEN LAST MEAL/SNACK AND BEDTIME: _____

NUMBER OF MEALS: _____ NUMBER OF SNACKS:_____

MINUTES OF EXERCISE: _____ LEVEL OF EXERCISE: _____

DAY 46

There is only one journey: going inside yourself.
                                    —Rainer Maria Rilke

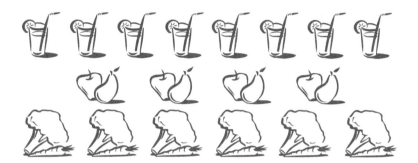

FAT GRAMS: _____ ALCOHOLIC BEVERAGES:_____

HOURS BETWEEN LAST MEAL/SNACK AND BEDTIME: _____

NUMBER OF MEALS: _____ NUMBER OF SNACKS:_____

MINUTES OF EXERCISE: _____ LEVEL OF EXERCISE: _____

DAY 47

He who, secure within, can say, tomorrow, do thy worst, for I have lived today.

—John Dryden

FAT GRAMS: _____ ALCOHOLIC BEVERAGES: _____

HOURS BETWEEN LAST MEAL/SNACK AND BEDTIME: _____

NUMBER OF MEALS: _____ NUMBER OF SNACKS: _____

MINUTES OF EXERCISE: _____ LEVEL OF EXERCISE: _____

DAY 48

When pain, betrayal, judgment, or adversity comes—I live that too. I can face it straight up and know that it, too, shall pass—every moment does.

—Oprah Winfrey

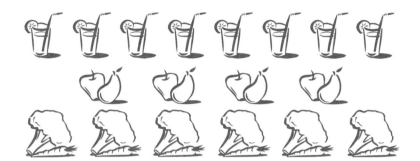

FAT GRAMS: _____ ALCOHOLIC BEVERAGES:_____

HOURS BETWEEN LAST MEAL/SNACK AND BEDTIME: _____

NUMBER OF MEALS: _____ NUMBER OF SNACKS:_____

MINUTES OF EXERCISE: _____ LEVEL OF EXERCISE: _____

DAY 49

It is not enough to do good; one must do it the right way.
—John, Viscount Morley of Blackburn

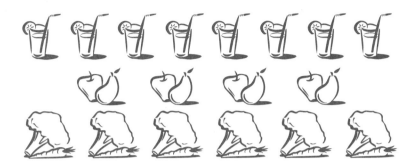

FAT GRAMS: _____ ALCOHOLIC BEVERAGES:_____

HOURS BETWEEN LAST MEAL/SNACK AND BEDTIME: _____

NUMBER OF MEALS: _____ NUMBER OF SNACKS:_____

MINUTES OF EXERCISE: _____ LEVEL OF EXERCISE: _____

_____

_____

_____

_____

_____

_____

_____

_____

DAY 50

We all need to accept and love ourselves no matter how we look. That means loving ourselves just as much now as when we reach our goal.

—Bob Greene

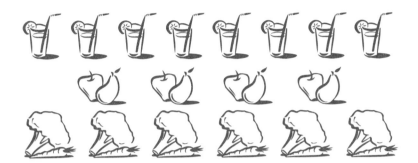

FAT GRAMS: _____ ALCOHOLIC BEVERAGES:_____

HOURS BETWEEN LAST MEAL/SNACK AND BEDTIME: _____

NUMBER OF MEALS: _____ NUMBER OF SNACKS:_____

MINUTES OF EXERCISE: _____ LEVEL OF EXERCISE: _____

TOTAL EXERCISE SESSIONS FOR THE PAST WEEK: _____ WEIGHT:_____

DAY 51

*If we had no winter, the spring would not be so pleasant;
if we did not sometimes taste of adversity, prosperity
would not be so welcome.*

—Anne Bradstreet

FAT GRAMS: _____ ALCOHOLIC BEVERAGES:_____

HOURS BETWEEN LAST MEAL/SNACK AND BEDTIME: _____

NUMBER OF MEALS: _____ NUMBER OF SNACKS:_____

MINUTES OF EXERCISE: _____ LEVEL OF EXERCISE: _____

DAY 52

Sometime in your life you will go on a journey. It will be the longest journey you have ever taken. It is the journey to find yourself.

—Katherine Sharp

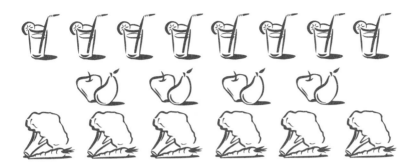

FAT GRAMS: _____ ALCOHOLIC BEVERAGES:_____

HOURS BETWEEN LAST MEAL/SNACK AND BEDTIME: _____

NUMBER OF MEALS: _____ NUMBER OF SNACKS:_____

MINUTES OF EXERCISE: _____ LEVEL OF EXERCISE: _____

DAY 53

Look after yourself every day and put forth your best effort to love yourself enough to do what's best.

—Oprah Winfrey

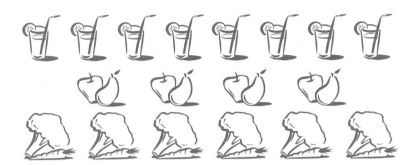

FAT GRAMS: _____   ALCOHOLIC BEVERAGES: _____

HOURS BETWEEN LAST MEAL/SNACK AND BEDTIME: _____

NUMBER OF MEALS: _____   NUMBER OF SNACKS: _____

MINUTES OF EXERCISE: _____   LEVEL OF EXERCISE: _____

_____

_____

_____

_____

_____

_____

_____

_____

DAY 54

I can't imagine a fulfilling life without the feeling of living in the moment and experiencing true joy.

—Bob Greene

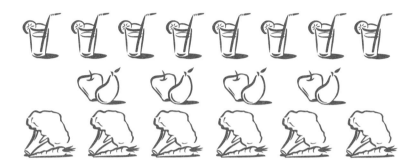

FAT GRAMS: _____ ALCOHOLIC BEVERAGES:_____

HOURS BETWEEN LAST MEAL/SNACK AND BEDTIME: _____

NUMBER OF MEALS: _____ NUMBER OF SNACKS:_____

MINUTES OF EXERCISE: _____ LEVEL OF EXERCISE: _____

_____

_____

_____

_____

_____

_____

_____

_____

DAY 55

To love oneself is the beginning of a lifelong romance.

—Oscar Wilde

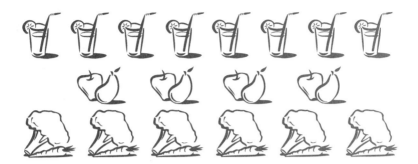

FAT GRAMS: _____ ALCOHOLIC BEVERAGES:_____

HOURS BETWEEN LAST MEAL/SNACK AND BEDTIME: _____

NUMBER OF MEALS: _____ NUMBER OF SNACKS:_____

MINUTES OF EXERCISE: _____ LEVEL OF EXERCISE: _____

_____

_____

_____

_____

_____

_____

_____

DAY 56

It is never too late to be what you might have been.

—George Eliot

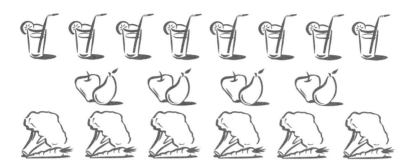

FAT GRAMS: _____ ALCOHOLIC BEVERAGES:_____

HOURS BETWEEN LAST MEAL/SNACK AND BEDTIME: _____

NUMBER OF MEALS: _____ NUMBER OF SNACKS:_____

MINUTES OF EXERCISE: _____ LEVEL OF EXERCISE: _____

DAY 57

Those who do not find the time for exercise will have to find time for illness.

—The earl of Derby

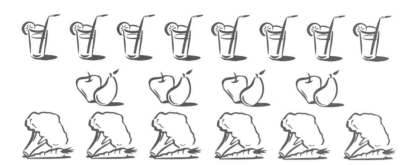

FAT GRAMS: _____ ALCOHOLIC BEVERAGES:_____

HOURS BETWEEN LAST MEAL/SNACK AND BEDTIME: _____

NUMBER OF MEALS: _____ NUMBER OF SNACKS:_____

MINUTES OF EXERCISE: _____ LEVEL OF EXERCISE: _____

TOTAL EXERCISE SESSIONS FOR THE PAST WEEK: _____ WEIGHT:_____

DAY 58

Always keep in mind that things happen, both good and bad, for a reason. There is always some life lesson in everything that happens to us. What's important is that we learn the lesson.

—Bob Greene

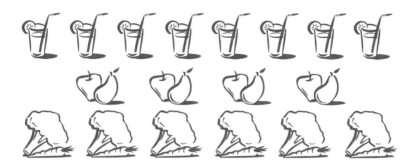

FAT GRAMS: _____ ALCOHOLIC BEVERAGES:_____

HOURS BETWEEN LAST MEAL/SNACK AND BEDTIME: _____

NUMBER OF MEALS: _____ NUMBER OF SNACKS:_____

MINUTES OF EXERCISE: _____ LEVEL OF EXERCISE: _____

DAY 59

Learning self-love takes time.

—Bob Greene

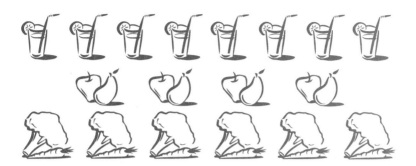

FAT GRAMS: _____ ALCOHOLIC BEVERAGES:_____

HOURS BETWEEN LAST MEAL/SNACK AND BEDTIME: _____

NUMBER OF MEALS: _____ NUMBER OF SNACKS:_____

MINUTES OF EXERCISE: _____ LEVEL OF EXERCISE: _____

_____

_____

_____

_____

_____

_____

_____

_____

DAY 60

All excellent things are as difficult as they are rare.
—Benedict Baruch Spinoza

FAT GRAMS: _____ ALCOHOLIC BEVERAGES:_____

HOURS BETWEEN LAST MEAL/SNACK AND BEDTIME: _____

NUMBER OF MEALS: _____ NUMBER OF SNACKS:_____

MINUTES OF EXERCISE: _____ LEVEL OF EXERCISE: _____

DAY 61

Until you make peace with who you are, you'll never be content with what you have.

—Doris Mortman

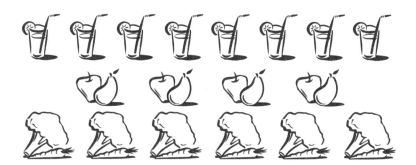

FAT GRAMS: _____ ALCOHOLIC BEVERAGES: _____

HOURS BETWEEN LAST MEAL/SNACK AND BEDTIME: _____

NUMBER OF MEALS: _____ NUMBER OF SNACKS: _____

MINUTES OF EXERCISE: _____ LEVEL OF EXERCISE: _____

DAY 62

Choice is the engine of our evolution.

—Gary Zukav

FAT GRAMS: _____ ALCOHOLIC BEVERAGES:_____

HOURS BETWEEN LAST MEAL/SNACK AND BEDTIME: _____

NUMBER OF MEALS: _____ NUMBER OF SNACKS:_____

MINUTES OF EXERCISE: _____ LEVEL OF EXERCISE: _____

_____

_____

_____

_____

_____

_____

_____

_____

DAY 63

You must understand that you create all that you are.

—Bob Greene

FAT GRAMS: _____ ALCOHOLIC BEVERAGES:_____

HOURS BETWEEN LAST MEAL/SNACK AND BEDTIME: _____

NUMBER OF MEALS: _____ NUMBER OF SNACKS:_____

MINUTES OF EXERCISE: _____ LEVEL OF EXERCISE: _____

DAY 64

You alone are responsible for your life.

—Oprah Winfrey

FAT GRAMS: _____ ALCOHOLIC BEVERAGES:_____

HOURS BETWEEN LAST MEAL/SNACK AND BEDTIME: _____

NUMBER OF MEALS: _____ NUMBER OF SNACKS:_____

MINUTES OF EXERCISE: _____ LEVEL OF EXERCISE: _____

TOTAL EXERCISE SESSIONS FOR THE PAST WEEK: _____ WEIGHT:_____

_____

_____

_____

_____

_____

_____

_____

DAY 65

We were born to make manifest the glory of God that is within.

—Marianne Williamson

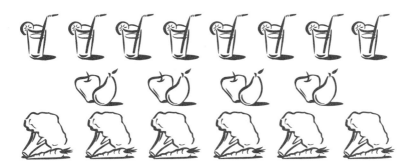

FAT GRAMS: _____ ALCOHOLIC BEVERAGES:_____

HOURS BETWEEN LAST MEAL/SNACK AND BEDTIME: _____

NUMBER OF MEALS: _____ NUMBER OF SNACKS:_____

MINUTES OF EXERCISE: _____ LEVEL OF EXERCISE: _____

DAY 66

We know the power is available to each of us, every moment of every day, but we have to ask that the spiritual switch be turned on. Next, we've got to be ready to bear the Glory.

—Sara Ban Breathnach

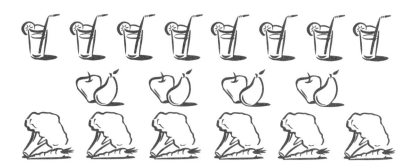

FAT GRAMS: _____ ALCOHOLIC BEVERAGES:_____

HOURS BETWEEN LAST MEAL/SNACK AND BEDTIME: _____

NUMBER OF MEALS: _____ NUMBER OF SNACKS:_____

MINUTES OF EXERCISE: _____ LEVEL OF EXERCISE: _____

_____

_____

_____

_____

_____

_____

_____

_____

DAY 67

Only after I experienced living in the moment was I able to experience true joy.

—Bob Greene

FAT GRAMS: _____ ALCOHOLIC BEVERAGES: _____

HOURS BETWEEN LAST MEAL/SNACK AND BEDTIME: _____

NUMBER OF MEALS: _____ NUMBER OF SNACKS: _____

MINUTES OF EXERCISE: _____ LEVEL OF EXERCISE: _____

DAY 68

True life is lived when small changes occur.

—Leo Tolstoy

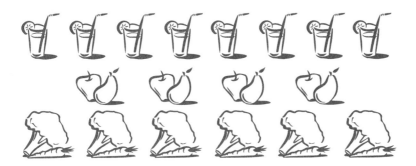

FAT GRAMS: _____ ALCOHOLIC BEVERAGES:_____

HOURS BETWEEN LAST MEAL/SNACK AND BEDTIME: _____

NUMBER OF MEALS: _____ NUMBER OF SNACKS:_____

MINUTES OF EXERCISE: _____ LEVEL OF EXERCISE: _____

_____

_____

_____

_____

_____

_____

_____

_____

DAY 69

Accepting yourself and living in the moment will together increase your opportunities for experiencing true joy. And when you have feelings of true joy on a regular basis, you are moving toward self-love. And that is a beautiful experience.

—Bob Greene

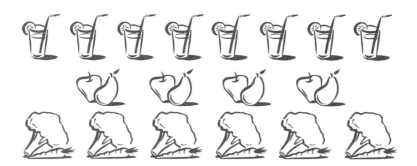

FAT GRAMS: _____ ALCOHOLIC BEVERAGES:_____

HOURS BETWEEN LAST MEAL/SNACK AND BEDTIME: _____

NUMBER OF MEALS: _____ NUMBER OF SNACKS:_____

MINUTES OF EXERCISE: _____ LEVEL OF EXERCISE: _____

DAY 70

True love begins with yourself.

—Oprah Winfrey

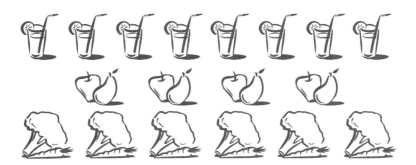

FAT GRAMS: _____ ALCOHOLIC BEVERAGES:_____

HOURS BETWEEN LAST MEAL/SNACK AND BEDTIME: _____

NUMBER OF MEALS: _____ NUMBER OF SNACKS:_____

MINUTES OF EXERCISE: _____ LEVEL OF EXERCISE: _____

DAY 71

If you want to find the answers to the Big Questions about your soul, you'd best begin with the Little Answers about your body.

–George Sheehan

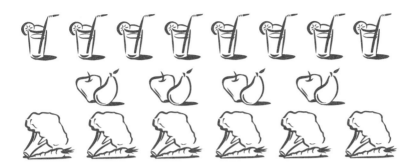

FAT GRAMS: _____ ALCOHOLIC BEVERAGES:_____

HOURS BETWEEN LAST MEAL/SNACK AND BEDTIME: _____

NUMBER OF MEALS: _____ NUMBER OF SNACKS:_____

MINUTES OF EXERCISE: _____ LEVEL OF EXERCISE: _____

TOTAL EXERCISE SESSIONS FOR THE PAST WEEK: _____ WEIGHT:_____

_____

_____

_____

_____

_____

_____

_____

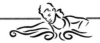

DAY 72

You gain strength, courage, and confidence by every experience in which you really stop to look fear in the face. . . . You must do the thing you cannot do.

—Eleanor Roosevelt

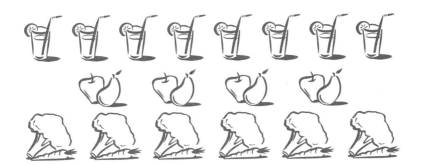

FAT GRAMS: _____   ALCOHOLIC BEVERAGES: _____

HOURS BETWEEN LAST MEAL/SNACK AND BEDTIME: _____

NUMBER OF MEALS: _____   NUMBER OF SNACKS: _____

MINUTES OF EXERCISE: _____   LEVEL OF EXERCISE: _____

_____

_____

_____

_____

_____

_____

_____

_____

DAY 73

I feel free. Free to live in the moment. Free to enjoy everyone I can.

—Oprah Winfrey

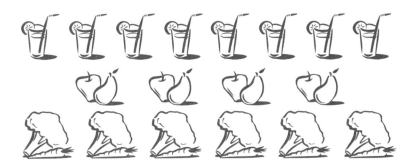

FAT GRAMS: _____ ALCOHOLIC BEVERAGES:_____

HOURS BETWEEN LAST MEAL/SNACK AND BEDTIME: _____

NUMBER OF MEALS: _____ NUMBER OF SNACKS:_____

MINUTES OF EXERCISE: _____ LEVEL OF EXERCISE: _____

DAY 74

When you are capable of self-love, you learn to love. To express love is our ultimate goal.

—Bob Greene

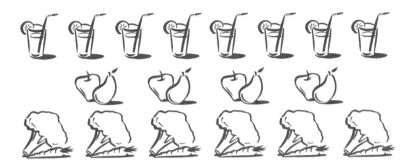

FAT GRAMS: _____ ALCOHOLIC BEVERAGES:_____

HOURS BETWEEN LAST MEAL/SNACK AND BEDTIME: _____

NUMBER OF MEALS: _____ NUMBER OF SNACKS:_____

MINUTES OF EXERCISE: _____ LEVEL OF EXERCISE: _____

DAY 75

There is only one happiness in life, to love and be loved.

—George Sand

FAT GRAMS: _____ ALCOHOLIC BEVERAGES:_____

HOURS BETWEEN LAST MEAL/SNACK AND BEDTIME: _____

NUMBER OF MEALS: _____ NUMBER OF SNACKS:_____

MINUTES OF EXERCISE: _____ LEVEL OF EXERCISE: _____

DAY 76

Nothing can bring you peace but yourself.
                                    −Ralph Waldo Emerson

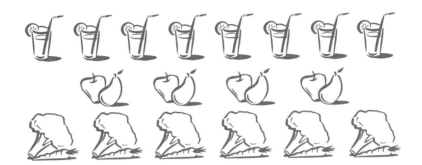

FAT GRAMS: _____ ALCOHOLIC BEVERAGES:_____

HOURS BETWEEN LAST MEAL/SNACK AND BEDTIME: _____

NUMBER OF MEALS: _____ NUMBER OF SNACKS:_____

MINUTES OF EXERCISE: _____ LEVEL OF EXERCISE: _____

DAY 77

Listening to your heart is not simple. Finding out who you are is not simple. It takes a lot of hard work and courage to get to know who you are and what you want.

—Sue Bender

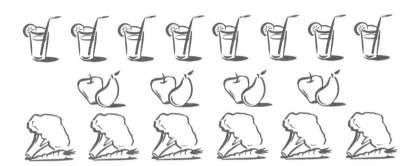

FAT GRAMS: _____ ALCOHOLIC BEVERAGES:_____

HOURS BETWEEN LAST MEAL/SNACK AND BEDTIME: _____

NUMBER OF MEALS: _____ NUMBER OF SNACKS:_____

MINUTES OF EXERCISE: _____ LEVEL OF EXERCISE: _____

DAY 78

It's the support and care and love that you give yourself that gives you the real strength to care for and love others.

—Oprah Winfrey

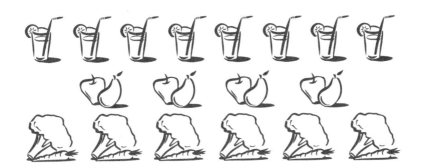

FAT GRAMS: _____ ALCOHOLIC BEVERAGES:_____

HOURS BETWEEN LAST MEAL/SNACK AND BEDTIME: _____

NUMBER OF MEALS: _____ NUMBER OF SNACKS:_____

MINUTES OF EXERCISE: _____ LEVEL OF EXERCISE: _____

TOTAL EXERCISE SESSIONS FOR THE PAST WEEK: _____ WEIGHT:_____

_____

_____

_____

_____

_____

_____

_____

DAY 79

Joy is not in things; it is in us.

—Richard Wagner

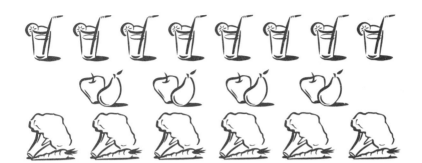

FAT GRAMS: _____ ALCOHOLIC BEVERAGES:_____

HOURS BETWEEN LAST MEAL/SNACK AND BEDTIME: _____

NUMBER OF MEALS: _____ NUMBER OF SNACKS:_____

MINUTES OF EXERCISE: _____ LEVEL OF EXERCISE: _____

_____

_____

_____

_____

_____

_____

_____

_____

DAY 80

Joy and sorrow are next-door neighbors.

—Proverb

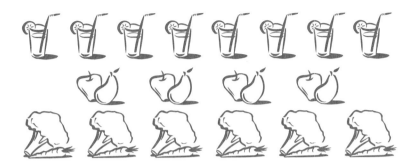

FAT GRAMS: _____ ALCOHOLIC BEVERAGES:_____

HOURS BETWEEN LAST MEAL/SNACK AND BEDTIME: _____

NUMBER OF MEALS: _____ NUMBER OF SNACKS:_____

MINUTES OF EXERCISE: _____ LEVEL OF EXERCISE: _____

DAY 81

Just remember that feeling sorrow and sadness will allow you to feel true joy to greater depths. Temporary setbacks are opportunities in disguise—opportunities to improve.

—Bob Greene

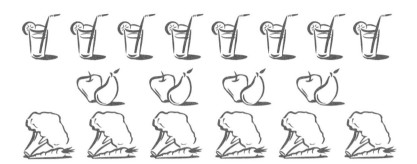

FAT GRAMS: _____ ALCOHOLIC BEVERAGES: _____

HOURS BETWEEN LAST MEAL/SNACK AND BEDTIME: _____

NUMBER OF MEALS: _____ NUMBER OF SNACKS: _____

MINUTES OF EXERCISE: _____ LEVEL OF EXERCISE: _____

_____

_____

_____

_____

_____

_____

_____

DAY 82

Learn to get in touch with the silence within yourself and know that everything in this life has a purpose.

—Elizabeth Kubler-Ross

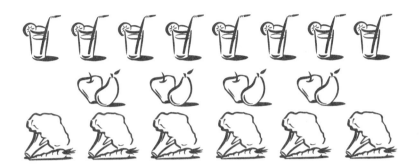

FAT GRAMS: _____ ALCOHOLIC BEVERAGES:_____

HOURS BETWEEN LAST MEAL/SNACK AND BEDTIME: _____

NUMBER OF MEALS: _____ NUMBER OF SNACKS:_____

MINUTES OF EXERCISE: _____ LEVEL OF EXERCISE: _____

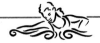

DAY 83

Inside myself is a place where I live all alone and that's where you renew your springs that never dry up.

—Pearl S. Buck

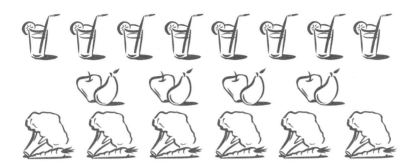

FAT GRAMS: _____ ALCOHOLIC BEVERAGES: _____

HOURS BETWEEN LAST MEAL/SNACK AND BEDTIME: _____

NUMBER OF MEALS: _____ NUMBER OF SNACKS: _____

MINUTES OF EXERCISE: _____ LEVEL OF EXERCISE: _____

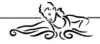

DAY 84

I can't stress enough the importance of living in the moment, of experiencing each moment, both the good and bad moments that make up your life. This will open you up to feelings of true joy, and that's what life is all about. After all, true joy is an expression of love.

— Bob Greene

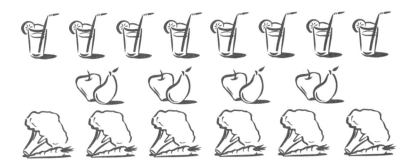

FAT GRAMS: _____ ALCOHOLIC BEVERAGES:_____

HOURS BETWEEN LAST MEAL/SNACK AND BEDTIME: _____

NUMBER OF MEALS: _____ NUMBER OF SNACKS:_____

MINUTES OF EXERCISE: _____ LEVEL OF EXERCISE: _____

DAY 85

Almost always it is the fear of being ourselves that brings us to the mirror.

—Antonio Porchia

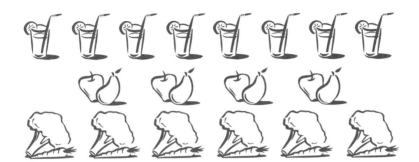

FAT GRAMS: _____ ALCOHOLIC BEVERAGES:_____

HOURS BETWEEN LAST MEAL/SNACK AND BEDTIME: _____

NUMBER OF MEALS: _____ NUMBER OF SNACKS:_____

MINUTES OF EXERCISE: _____ LEVEL OF EXERCISE: _____

TOTAL EXERCISE SESSIONS FOR THE PAST WEEK: _____ WEIGHT:_____

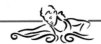

DAY 86

Everything in life that we really accept undergoes a change.

—Katherine Mansfield

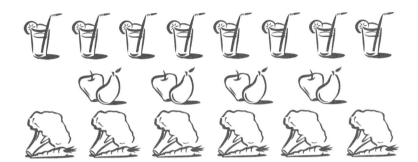

FAT GRAMS: _____ ALCOHOLIC BEVERAGES: _____

HOURS BETWEEN LAST MEAL/SNACK AND BEDTIME: _____

NUMBER OF MEALS: _____ NUMBER OF SNACKS: _____

MINUTES OF EXERCISE: _____ LEVEL OF EXERCISE: _____

_____

_____

_____

_____

_____

_____

_____

_____

_____

DAY 87

When we truly care for ourselves, it becomes possible to care far more profoundly about other people. The more alert and sensitive we are to our own needs, the more loving and generous we can be toward others.

—Eda LeShan

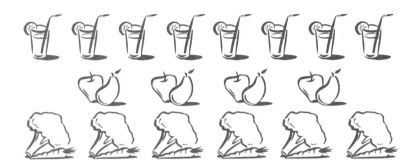

FAT GRAMS: _____ ALCOHOLIC BEVERAGES:_____

HOURS BETWEEN LAST MEAL/SNACK AND BEDTIME: _____

NUMBER OF MEALS: _____ NUMBER OF SNACKS:_____

MINUTES OF EXERCISE: _____ LEVEL OF EXERCISE: _____

_____

_____

_____

_____

_____

_____

_____

_____

DAY 88

It's difficult to change your habits—and ultimately your life. But you can do it.

—Bob Greene

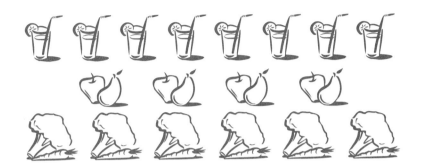

FAT GRAMS: _____ ALCOHOLIC BEVERAGES: _____

HOURS BETWEEN LAST MEAL/SNACK AND BEDTIME: _____

NUMBER OF MEALS: _____ NUMBER OF SNACKS: _____

MINUTES OF EXERCISE: _____ LEVEL OF EXERCISE: _____

DAY 89

There are no riches above a sound body.

—Ecclesiasticus 30:16

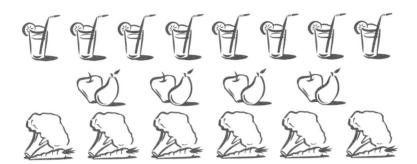

FAT GRAMS: _____ ALCOHOLIC BEVERAGES:_____

HOURS BETWEEN LAST MEAL/SNACK AND BEDTIME: _____

NUMBER OF MEALS: _____ NUMBER OF SNACKS:_____

MINUTES OF EXERCISE: _____ LEVEL OF EXERCISE: _____

_____

_____

_____

_____

_____

_____

_____

_____

DAY 90

It is good to have an end to journey towards; but it is the journey that matters in the end.

—Ursula K. LeGuin

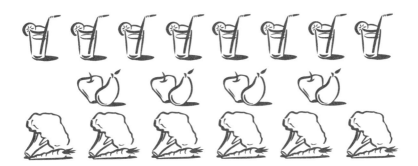

FAT GRAMS: _____ ALCOHOLIC BEVERAGES:_____

HOURS BETWEEN LAST MEAL/SNACK AND BEDTIME: _____

NUMBER OF MEALS: _____ NUMBER OF SNACKS:_____

MINUTES OF EXERCISE: _____ LEVEL OF EXERCISE: _____

_____

_____

_____

_____

_____

_____

_____

_____

_____

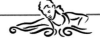

DAY 91

Possess your soul with patience.

—John Dryden

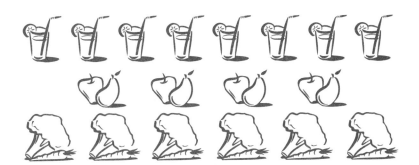

FAT GRAMS: _____ ALCOHOLIC BEVERAGES:_____

HOURS BETWEEN LAST MEAL/SNACK AND BEDTIME: _____

NUMBER OF MEALS: _____ NUMBER OF SNACKS:_____

MINUTES OF EXERCISE: _____ LEVEL OF EXERCISE: _____

_____

_____

_____

_____

_____

_____

_____

_____

DAY 92

I'm no longer afraid. I am more connected to myself.

—Oprah Winfrey

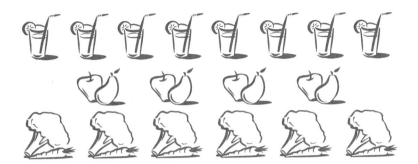

FAT GRAMS: _____ ALCOHOLIC BEVERAGES:_____

HOURS BETWEEN LAST MEAL/SNACK AND BEDTIME: _____

NUMBER OF MEALS: _____ NUMBER OF SNACKS:_____

MINUTES OF EXERCISE: _____ LEVEL OF EXERCISE: _____

TOTAL EXERCISE SESSIONS FOR THE PAST WEEK: _____ WEIGHT:_____